CW01336483

Journey through Pudendal Neuralgia

*Learning to live with
Pelvic Nerve Pain*

Margaret Stubbs

AuthorHouse™
1663 Liberty Drive
Bloomington, IN 47403
www.authorhouse.com
Phone: 1-800-839-8640

© 2011 Margaret Stubbs. All rights reserved.

No part of this book may be reproduced, stored in a retrieval system, or transmitted by any means without the written permission of the author.

First published by AuthorHouse 5/23/2011

ISBN: 978-1-4567-7372-4 (sc)

Printed in the United States of America

Any people depicted in stock imagery provided by Thinkstock are models, and such images are being used for illustrative purposes only. Certain stock imagery © Thinkstock.

This book is printed on acid-free paper.

Because of the dynamic nature of the Internet, any web addresses or links contained in this book may have changed since publication and may no longer be valid. The views expressed in this work are solely those of the author and do not necessarily reflect the views of the publisher, and the publisher hereby disclaims any responsibility for them.

Contents

Chapter 1 - Introduction	1
Chapter 2 – Personal Journey	4
Chapter 3 - Emotional Challenges	18
The Way Forward	20
Chapter 4 - Pudendal Neuralgia: What it is and how is it caused?	22
Definition	22
Symptoms and Diagnosis	23
Symptoms	23
Diagnosis	25
Chapter 5 - Treatments	27
Drug Therapy	27
Nerve Block Interventions	33
Pain Psychology	36
Physiotherapy	38
Decompression Surgery	42
Sacral Root Stimulation	43
Botox Injections	45
Research	45
Chapter 6 - Chronic Pain versus Acute Pain	46
Chapter 7 - Aids to Assist Normal Living	50
Chapter 8 - Conclusion	53
Helpful websites	55
References	56

Journey through Pudendal Neuralgia

Chapter 1 -
Introduction

"Pudendal Neuralgia" said the specialist at the end of my hour-long appointment, on the 1st October 2009. To most people this would be a very strange sounding term and to many it means absolutely nothing. However, it is a very distressing nerve pain condition, which seems very difficult to treat, and for which there currently seems to be no complete cure. The more I have learnt about it, the more depressing it might seem, not only that, but with its very situation in the body, for both men and women in the perineal area, it is also a rather embarrassing condition to discuss, especially with people of the opposite sex. Prior to this appointment, I had for some months wondered if this was the condition I was suffering from, but until this time, no one had been able to give my pain a name.

I have been suffering from what I believe is a form of chronic pelvic nerve pain for approximately two and a half years now. On the Internet there are only a few abstracts from journals in the field, but actually there seems to be very little written on this particular problem. For the sufferer it means it is a real challenge to find any books that can be used to help or guide. For this very reason, as a health professional myself seeking to come to terms with long term nerve pain, I felt it vital to try and remedy this state of affairs so that others like myself would have somewhere to turn for help and advice. I am not seeking to give definitive advice about the way forward, nor am I trying to be too clinical in the way I explain the problem. My aim is to use my own story to assist others in their search for ways to manage this pain, and to encourage all who go through this to keep trying the various options and asking for the necessary referrals, so that hopefully you can find treatments that may help.

In doing this I want to include other peoples' knowledge and experiences, so that I can give a balanced and more accurate approach to what is happening in the world at large as far as the treatment and management of pelvic nerve pain is concerned and what the future holds for us. I will use my own personal journey to set the scene, before providing practical ways forward that I hope will benefit many. I have included a list of helpful websites at the end as a resource for those of you who do not know where to turn for help. I know that there are so many others out there like myself, who are struggling to come to terms with a pain without pathology, i.e. one that has no apparent physical cause, who sometimes feel that they must be going mad, because the pain is so strange and so hard to explain to others.

I hope to be able to answer the questions, which many of us ask, so that carers and sufferers alike may be able to gain a more comprehensive insight into this condition, and thereby be able to manage the condition and be able to obtain the best out of life and not feel permanently limited by it.

Chronic pain is currently being brought to the attention of both government and medical organisations and the Chronic Pain Policy Coalition (www.paincoalition.org.uk) is working hard to have pain recognised as a disease in itself. 7.8 million people in the UK are currently suffering from chronic pain of some form, and 25% of those will lose their jobs as a result and 22% will suffer also from depression.

The coalition is working to address the issues of pain, so that more government funding is available to help manage and treat chronic pain. This is so that those of us who are affected in this way can have a realistic opportunity of being able to work, and are not forced to give up all our personal aspirations and independence. The Pelvic Pain Support Network, of which I am a member, is a supporter of the Chronic Pain Policy Coalition. Health Professionals, patient and industry representatives are all working in this coalition to establish pain on the healthcare agenda. So, those of you reading this, who may at times despair, in time things will change and we need to support the effort to bring that about.

Chapter 2 –
Personal Journey

It is hard to know where to begin, when looking back over the past few years and all that has happened. What is quite apparent is that the onset of this nerve pain has changed the direction of my life, in a way that I could not have anticipated and at times I find it hard to come to terms with. My pain journey has so far covered about two and a half years, which seems a long time to me, however I realise that this is a comparatively short length of time compared to a large proportion of sufferers, who may have been struggling with this condition for 10 or more years.

In July 2008, I was on holiday with my family in France, enjoying the weather and scenery there, when I had what appeared to be cystitis. On return to the UK I saw my GP and was prescribed antibiotics; it was my first ever experience of cystitis, but it was to be unforgettable. It didn't matter what I was treated with, I had constant bladder pain, and my GP quickly realized that this was not a usual form of cystitis. This could not be effectively treated with antibiotics and so I was referred to an urologist (who will remain nameless), who put me through some very undignified tests, but basically told me I had an overactive bladder.

As the situation did not improve, I obtained a second opinion from another urologist, who recognized the symptoms immediately and told me that if I had a cystoscopy with a urethral stretch and 6 weeks of antibiotics, I would never have any more problems, I'd feel fine within a week.

Sadly, he was wrong and the converse has been the case; within a week of having this minor bladder procedure, I found I could not sit for long periods, and sitting in the car became particularly challenging, I felt as if there was a lump in my vagina and it was unbearable. Apart from anything else this was an incredibly distressing pain to describe to others, particularly to any male friends. I kept going back to my urologist over the next 2 -3 months. Firstly, having tried the surgery, he then tried a steroid injection into my urethra, (thinking the problem was caused by an inflamed urethra); at the same time I started to try a variety of analgesic drugs, using my own knowledge to guide me. The urologist even organized an Magnetic Resonance Imaging (MRI) scan to rule out any other pathology, but no abnormalities were found.

He kept asking me if my pain was urethral pain? How does one know what is "urethral pain", I really had no idea? I just knew the pain was different to any pain I had ever experienced before and felt like it was right inside me, and that there was a lump sitting just inside my bladder or vagina, and I could no longer sit comfortably on any ordinary chair or seat (apart from a toilet seat).

In those first 6 weeks or so following the surgery, the pain did not improve and in fact brought some strange limitations to aspects of my life, which have remained as part of my life. In terms of what clothes I could wear I found that I could no longer wear either fitted trousers or tights, as they aggravated the pain, and were quite distressing, feeling as though I was being cut in two along my perineum. Even underwear could cause quite a significant discomfort.

I continued to find that sitting for long periods was virtually impossible, so car journeys of more than an hour were best avoided, and going to the cinema or theatre was out of the question, and as for cycling, well forget it. It also had a very dampening effect on (my) sex life, as the whole region was so hypersensitive to touch and so actual intercourse became much less frequent. I kept trying to return to work my regular hours but it was a struggle, and it was not until around Christmas that I eventually attempted to build up my hours again. In fact I was never able to work the 26 hours that were in my contract again, following the onset of this pain. As the pain tends to deteriorate as the days goes on, long hours at work often prove quite challenging.

The pain/discomfort has always been hard to describe, because it is not like other pain (nociceptive pain). For me, the pain does not stab, throb, ache, rather it is like an internal soreness, bruising, rubbing, burning, searing, tingling or prickling which can get incredibly intense and can give the sensation of having a lump in the vaginal area, or that you are sitting on something in the vaginal or vulval area. This has been my experience of this pain so far, but it can vary so much from person to person, as this pain like any other is rather subjective.

Initially the pain could waken me during the night, probably due to the more acute nociceptive element but now it no longer does as seems typical of this particular type of nerve pain.

At this time my middle daughter was studying pain in her Neurology module of her Biomedical Science Degree course, and had come home for the Christmas holiday. As we discussed the problem I was experiencing, we came to the conclusion that I was in fact suffering from "nerve pain". As a result when I saw my urologist in the New Year we discussed our findings with him, and he agreed we were probably right. He made the decision that I should start taking Amitryptiline, which is known to be effective in dealing with pelvic type nerve pain.

At this time I also browsed on the Internet and looked at a number of web sites, which had some information on nerve pain of this nature. They seemed to be describing my symptoms, so it confirmed to me what was going on. Various treatments were described there including different nerve blocks and, certain drug therapies. I also tried looking in the library and bookshops to see if there were any publications concerning pelvic nerve pain, and to date, I have found very few. It seems to be an area about which little is known particularly among the lay population, and treatments are rather uncertain.

Unfortunately, although I could tolerate 10mg/day of the Amitryptiline, when I increased the dose to 25 mg, I developed an allergic response, with a very itchy rash all over the trunk of my body, which did not subside even if I took a regular antihistamine. My GP advised me to stop, and started me on Pregabalin, another drug used often to treat Diabetic Neuropathy. This drug seemed to have strange side effects, and I was unable to tolerate more than 100mg/day; even then my sleep was now frequently broken at night, I felt quite queasy a lot of the time, found it harder to concentrate and if I tried adding in a pain killer such as Tramadol, I would almost fall asleep 24 hours after taking it. When I tried to increase the dose of Pregabalin, I was barely able to function, my legs felt so heavy I could barely walk, my thinking and reactions became very slow, and I felt incredibly nauseated.

At the same time, this drug had almost no beneficial effects at all on the pain. The nerve pain did not go away and some days I could hardly do anything due to the pain and could not tolerate more than 50mg Tramadol /day (which would knock the pain on the head for a few hours). Having tried to return to work after 6 weeks off sick, I struggled with my working hours, and consistently kept my working hours to 6 hours/day instead of the 8.5hours/day, which I had been used to.

By April (6 months after the pain first appeared) I felt I needed to find some expert help to assist with managing the pain, due to the distinct lack of progress, and persuaded my urologist to refer me to a local pain management consultant, who had been recommended to me and whom I could see privately (thanks to the insurance cover provided by my husband's employers). In him I found someone who understood my symptoms, although he wasn't exactly sure which nerves were causing the problem. Under his care I firstly had an epidural and an inguinal nerve block. There seemed to me to be little change in my pain and symptoms in the weeks that followed, so he then decided to carry out a Ganglion Impar block, where a steroid was injected onto the Ganglion impar (a collection of nerve cells lying just outside the spinal cord). Sadly, although there was a very slight improvement, it didn't last, but he believed the next course of action would be to stun the nerves in the Ganglion impar; this is called radiofrequency de-nervation. I wish he hadn't bothered, as this only stirred the pain up more, immediately after I went home.

The latter procedure was only performed, because he thought I was desperate for some improvement, and when it appeared to add no benefit, he referred me to a specialist in London who specialized in Uro-Genital pain (I tend to refer to it as 'Pelvic nerve pain"- as it seems a more acceptable way of talking about it). Before he referred me, I asked him, if he thought my problem was Pudendal Neuralgia, but he thought not, as he didn't think that the symptoms I had described to him matched up with that diagnosis.

On our summer holiday in 2009, we knew there could be no cycling, but as we were staying in the Algarve and it was beautifully warm, swimming was the best option. Unfortunately, after just a few days, I became aware that wet swim wear made the nerve pain worse, and so I could not sit in the sun having just come out of the swimming pool, I had to keep changing my bikini bottoms. Even then, I had lots of discomfort, and although I was very relaxed, the pain did not settle, but in fact seemed to deteriorate. I have since learnt that swimming breast - stroke, can make the pain worse- something I was unaware of at the time, and this obviously added to the problem.

It was then September, and I had been unable to return to my normal working hours since the initial surgery, almost a year earlier, and was finding life very challenging. My employers who had in the early months of the year been very understanding and supportive, seemed to have moved in their stance towards me, and I now felt under intense pressure to perform, and in order to manage my work better

I had started doing my administrative work from home to enable me to cope with the practical side of my role.

By this stage I was now beginning to wonder if life would ever return to normal, after all what was normal now? I couldn't manage my regular working day and I was unable to take on much in the evenings, because by that time of day, the pain was often at its worst. The only way I have been able to maintain any semblance of normality, is due to a very kind friend who made a foam ring cushion for me, (just a month or so after the pain first kicked in), so that I could sit for longer as the pressure was taken off the most sensitive areas. With this I could sit through a church service and go to the band of which I was a member. I still couldn't participate in some of the concerts, because I could not cope with the length of time spent in the car on top of the concert itself.

Over this period of time I really felt that I had made no improvement at all, and wondered if this nerve pain would ever come to an end. I was quite relieved to be referred to this particular specialist, as having looked on the internet, I found he was one of the key experts in this field in the UK as far as I could see. My first appointment was to be an hour long, in order that he could discern the problem and make the correct diagnosis. I was advised to have someone to accompany me and as my husband works in London, he agreed to meet me there.

I knew this might be a difficult appointment, because knowing the location of the nerve pain, I was aware that there might be potentially embarrassing questions asked in the process. It was just as I imagined, and within a few minutes of being in the consulting room, I was being shown a diagram of a woman's vulval anatomy and asked to point out where the pain occurred. I was also questioned as to whether opening bowels, having sexual intercourse or passing urine triggered the onset of pain. All of these can trigger painful episodes. Up until this occasion no one had ever suggested a vaginal examination, but that day this also was on the cards, in order to pinpoint what triggered the pain. The upshot of this was that he gave a name to the problem, which fitted with my own perception of what was happening. He said that from his examination, the history I had given, where I felt the pain, and the nature of the trigger factors, he believed that I probably had Pudendal Neuralgia.

He was not specific about why it had started, although he wondered if the original bladder pain was part of the same problem and that surgery could have triggered the pain, as this is one of the classic risk factors. However I was surprised that my having been a fairly keen cyclist didn't seem to concern him much (although, so much of what I had read on various websites indicated that this was often called "cyclist's syndrome"). Like me he did not think that the small dose of Pregabalin that I was taking was helping, so told me I could gradually reduce the dose and then withdraw from taking it, which delighted me.

My own interpretation of the situation is this, that my cycling has probably made me more susceptible to this kind of nerve injury, maybe even damaging or compressing the nerves during the prolonged periods of time I have been cycling. I had been cycling fairly regularly ever since I was about eleven. I have also had three children, all born by a normal vaginal delivery, which can impact the pudendal nerves. Then, the bladder surgery probably irritated or damaged the nerve still further, so that now I was experiencing this type of nerve pain.

Various treatment options were suggested and so within a week I had undergone my first bilateral pudendal nerve block at the level of the ischial spine. I hardly noticed any change, so a month later I had a second. As this appeared not to bring about any improvement, we (the consultant and I) then discussed the way forward. He decided to do one further Pudendal Nerve Block at the level of the ischial spine and then after that, if there was no change I should undergo a block lower down the nerve at the level of Alcock's canal, by means of a Computerized Tomography scan (CT scan). All these nerve blocks were done under sedation. I have since been informed that there are other experts who believe that the patient should be fully awake during the procedure, as they believe it is important that the patient is fully alert to assess the pain level immediately following the nerve block. As with many things in life, there are contrasting opinions on what is the best or safest method.

By this time (late November) I had stopped taking the Pregabalin, and had started Duloxetine 30mg daily to give me better relief over the Christmas period until the block under CT scan. I found the Duloxetine made me feel very nauseated straight away and so having started taking it every day, I initially reduced it to alternate days. Then I started taking an anti emetic to try and relieve the nausea, so increased the dose of Duloxetine back to a daily dose of 30mg. However, after 2 weeks of struggling even with an anti –emetic, I was forced to reduce the Duloxetine back to alternate days to try and manage the nausea. When I was taking it every day, it seemed to have a beneficial effect on the nerve pain, and the pain was much easier to live with.

Unfortunately, there was no way that I could maintain a daily dose, without losing weight due to the nausea affecting my appetite. By reducing the Duloxetine to alternate days, the pain started to come back, although not with the same intensity. As I continued with alternate days, the pain increased, so I decided to try two days out of three, at the same time as I started on a new brand of Duloxetine, which increased the level of nausea again.

I had the third nerve block in December, with no change to the pain levels. I was then booked for the block under CT scan. I found this more difficult, as I had got used to the standard procedure of climbing onto the theatre table and lying face down for the injections into my buttocks, (although it has to be said that I still always felt rather exposed and vulnerable in this position). The CT scan was far worse, as I had to basically lie face down on this couch in the CT scanner, with my gown undone and my buttocks exposed while the scan was done and the exact position for these injections marked on my buttocks. It was at this point that I came to the conclusion that I did not want any more of this kind of treatment. If there were some improvement to be gained then I felt I could cope with going through the indignity of it all, but if the outcome showed no improvement, then I felt it would be preferable not to have that type of nerve block again. In fact there was no noticeable change for the better following the first nerve block via Alcock's canal.

At this point I then spent a significant amount of time researching much more intensely on the Internet, on the subject of Pudendal Neuralgia, the treatments available, the success rates and realized that there was probably nothing more in the way of nerve blocks that could now be done. I had tried a variety of medications recommended and endorsed by The National Institute for Health and Clinical Excellence (NICE) for neuropathic pain, and had found one that helped, as long as I could manage the side effects from it.

I then carefully researched the topic of nerve decompression surgery, for which the rate of recovery seemed incredibly slow to me, taking two to three years sometimes to make any significant difference. However, through the Pelvic Pain Support Network (www.pelvicpain.org.uk), I learnt that a fair number of people who had undergone surgery in France felt that their pain had improved significantly in the long term and that as their pain had been so severe prior to the surgery, and their quality of life so poor, they felt the surgery was well worth it. It appeared that in the UK there was only one surgeon who carried out this type of surgery. The current centre of excellence for this surgery is in Nantes in France, where a team has been working in this field for about 25 years, and where certain approaches to this surgery have been pioneered. This centre has also published the only randomized controlled surgical trial into surgical decompression of the pudendal nerves.

Through the Pelvic Pain Support Network message board I discovered there to be quite a number of other people with similar nerve pain problems and this was where I asked my many questions about decompression surgery. No one at any point ever suggested the problem could be completely cured and I started to wonder if there was still any hope of me gaining any significant improvement.

As I had to see my consultant again to discuss the way forward, I planned to enquire about the feasibility of surgery for me. Very early in this consultation, before I had asked a single question, he informed me, that judging from the lack of response to Pudendal nerve blocks, both at Ischial spine level and also Alcock's canal level, it was more than likely that my nerves would not respond positively to surgery, as they were probably already too badly damaged.

When I exchanged experiences with other patients, they suggested that because this had been my experience, surgery did not need to be ruled out. Some other patients had been through similar experiences, yet when the nerve blocks had been performed in France they had experienced some relief albeit temporary and they had later undergone surgery. However, it has to be said that this form of treatment comes at a significant cost financially, unless one is able to obtain funding on the National Health Service (NHS), which is generally quite hard to do.

As surgery does not now appear to be an option, and also I was keen to try less invasive measures first, I then transferred to the NHS and the Pain Management Centre at the National Hospital for Neurology and Neurosurgery (London) for a possible trial of Sacral Root Stimulation (a form of Spinal Cord Stimulation). This could only take place if my Local Primary Care Trust (PCT) were prepared to fund the treatment (Spinal Cord Stimulation is a NICE approved treatment for pain management). In the meantime, I have had to balance out the nerve pain with the drugs available to me at the moment, and keep on with as many of my activities as I can. I had an appointment to discuss the possibility of this option in June and was waiting for a trial of Sacral Root Stimulation in November 2010.

However, in the meantime following the recommendation of a friend with Pudendal Neuralgia, I started a course of physiotherapy treatment with a physiotherapist who specialised in treating pelvic pain. This includes manual therapy and trigger point therapy and uses the process of biofeedback to help improve both contraction and relaxation of the pelvic floor. This now appears to have brought improvement, as I have been able to reduce the amount of pain relief that I take and can manage the pain better with the use of a Transcutaneous Nerve Stimulation (TENS) machine. I have now withdrawn from having the Sacral Root Stimulation programme, because I have learnt to manage this pain using several prescribed drugs and a TENS machine.

The fact is now, that for whatever reason, I have chronic nerve pain in the form of Pudendal Neuralgia, and whilst it is not a life threatening condition, it is life limiting and I must accept the associated limitations and look for new opportunities out of this. It has changed the direction of my career, and has made me review my priorities in life quite drastically. Out of this I want to try and help anyone else who has ever, or is now experiencing similar pain to myself. I want to encourage others to seek opportunities for treatment and to offer support to others. I would like to believe that good can be brought out of a difficult situation, and so want to offer this as a resource for fellow sufferers.

Every so often during the first 12 months, there were periods of 3-4 days when the pain was minimal and then I wondered if this was the start of my recovery. However, these have never lasted longer than that and then the pain has always come back, often with a vengeance. For me coming back to the UK after my summer holiday in the sun in (2009), it was so disappointing to know that the pain had deteriorated during the holiday, when all hopes had been set on an improvement.

Being able to adapt to having long- term pain is a significant challenge and not easy to come to terms with, albeit I have only had the pain for approximately two and a half years. Even now, I am only just beginning to accept that I may only be able to work a limited number of hours a day and that I possibly will not achieve what I might previously have hoped for in terms of a career. However, I have a loving and supportive husband and family, and have discovered some wonderful friends, who have not given up on me, and am learning so much about myself through my responses to long- term pain.

Chapter 3 -
Emotional Challenges

There are a number of aspects of this current nerve pain condition that have challenged me emotionally. One is the very nature of the pain; who would want to talk about a pain that comes from such a personal area; this has made it difficult at times to share what it is like. Another is how to describe nerve pain and also the effect of nerve pain on one's emotions. On occasions I have been reduced to tears, I do not know what to do with myself. At times I cannot bear sitting or standing anymore, so have to yet again go and lie down on my bed and hope things improve. How can anyone understand how clothing makes the problem worse, and that I cannot bear to have trousers on for any length of time, or tights, or the necessity of having to buy special underwear without seams, for days when the pain is unbearable.

How does one speak of the frustration of not being able to enjoy normal sexual intimacy, due to the strange sensations one experiences in the perineal and vulval areas and the side effects of drugs, which reduce sexual enjoyment? Unless a person has prior experience, they can have no concept of what nerve pain is all about, and I was one of those until about two and a half years ago. The fact there is no outright cure for this and most treatments do not even promise more than a little improvement, is depressing in itself. The pain makes driving anywhere a nightmare, so this limits any work that involves driving very much. What work is actually possible when one cannot predict the pain levels by the end of the day, as the pain normally increases during the course of a day?

Chronic pain does not happen in isolation, we each have a personality, things we like and dislike (4therapy.com 2010), When we experience long term pain it affects every part of us and can complicate our lives, so that we no longer behave as we used to, we feel more stressed, relationships with friends and family can break down, we finder it harder to cope both emotionally and physically. As I said a little earlier, the nature of this pain has left me at times feeling isolated as I struggle to explain the nature of this pain to others. I have felt quite depressed at times and am sure I am not alone in this, at other times I have been angry at what has happened.

I believe that depression is more than just a possibility with this debilitating condition, and I would urge all sufferers to acknowledge that they need emotional support, either through medication, Cognitive Behavioural Therapy, counselling, or whatever helps them as an individual.

For me this all got too much by summer 2009, 8 months after the pain first started, and I asked my GP for antidepressants, unfortunately the dose he gave me interacted with the Pregabalin I was then taking, and I felt drunk all the time, very sick, lightheaded and unable to think straight, so I decided to stop after a week of this and see how things went. However, by December the stress of trying to fulfil my role at work and prove to my employers that I could cope and also manage with the ongoing pain was overwhelming and I knew that I either had to quit work or take anti depressants. Initially I went for the latter, but just one month later I had resigned.

For 6 months I took a tablet (Duloxetine) that combats both the depression and the nerve pain, but which I could only seem to tolerate 2 out of 3 days. I took the equivalent of 20mg/day, not a therapeutic dose for either depression or nerve pain, but better than nothing, and with the addition of Tramadol, I could cope with a significantly reduced level of pain

The Way Forward

What does the future hold? Will I be able to hold down a fulfilling job? Will life ever be normal again? Will sex ever be what it was; thank goodness I have a very loving and understanding husband, who has been infinitely patient during this time?

The condition has made me feel very vulnerable on occasions, and so has the treatment. It seems there is no longer anything very much that is private now.

For me a real break through came, when I found the Pelvic Pain Support Network on the Internet. When I e-mailed for more information, I was so encouraged to receive a telephone with someone from the network. Suddenly, I had come into contact with another person who understood my pain issues. I then registered to use the message board and have found that to be a very helpful place to go for advice, suggestions and support with various challenging issues. This support network has become so helpful to me and I would encourage anyone suffering with any type of pelvic pain with or without a definite diagnosis, to make contact with this network. There are so many other people who are going through similar experiences, or have been through similar experiences and are further down the road and can help those of us less familiar with the different ways to try and manage chronic pain. I have developed a couple of friendships with fellow sufferers, through contact with others who use this network.

As I said a little earlier, I was waiting for a possible trial of a sacral root Stimulator; (similar to Spinal Cord Stimulation). However, following recommendations from two fellow pelvic pain sufferers, I tried some specialist physiotherapy. I tried manual therapy, to see if it would help my condition. I can now see that there might be some light at the end of the tunnel, and that improvement is possible.

The importance of a multi disciplinary approach to treatment cannot be underestimated. All the therapies that I am going to describe are part of the provision of holistic care to those who suffer with this particular form of chronic pain. Psychologists and physiotherapists are part of this team and work alongside the pain management consultant to provide the care required to help the individual live with their pain. Each sufferer is an individual and will have different responses to the various aspects of treatment offered, but it is important to try them and hopefully find some form of relief at some point and ways to manage the pain.

Chapter 4 -
Pudendal Neuralgia: What it is and how is it caused?

Definition

Pudendal neuralgia is a painful neuropathic condition, caused by inflammation of the pudendal nerve. It is a disorder of the pudendal nerve that can lead to chronic nerve pain.

Pudendal neuralgia (also known as Pudendal Canal Syndrome, Alcock's Canal Syndrome, Cyclist's Syndrome and Pudendal Nerve Entrapment, PNE) is a form of nerve pain (neuropathy, neuritis) where the symptoms are perceived to be in the pelvis / pelvic / perineal region (genitals, perianal).

The pudendal nerve runs through the buttocks (gluteus muscles) and into the perineum (the part of the body touching a cycle saddle), this includes the vulva, vagina and anus in women, and penis, scrotum and anus in men.

Causes

There are thought to be a variety of possible causes; Prolonged and heavy cycling on an inappropriately shaped or incorrectly positioned bicycle saddle.

Diabetic neuropathy

Trauma to the perineal area (episiotomy, forceps delivery), pelvis and buttocks- including childbirth, fracture to the pelvis or blunt trauma (straddle injury)

- Excessive sitting
- Horse riding
- Sitting at a computer constantly
- Thickening of ligaments around the pudendal nerve
- Bony formations pushing against the pudendal nerve
- Chronic constipation
- Pelvic surgery

Symptoms and Diagnosis

Symptoms

The pelvic pain is worsened by sitting and may be relieved by lying down); it can include prickling, stabbing, burning, numbness, and the sense of a foreign object in the urethra, penis or vagina, and rectum. In addition to pain, sexual dysfunction, impotence, faecal and urinary incontinence can be a problem.

Pain may present in any of the following ways:

- Pain in the perineum or anal region

- In men, pain in the penis or scrotum
- In women, pain in the labia or vulva (vulvodynia)
- Pain during/after sexual intercourse
- Pain during/after urinating or having a bowel movement
- Pain which comes on when sitting, relieved by standing

Initially symptoms may be one sided but can be present on both sides as time progresses

- With or without touch
- In men, this may appear as pain during erection, difficulty sustaining erection or painful ejaculation.

Other symptoms may include:

- Difficulty in urination/ defaecation
- Urinary hesitation, urgency and or frequency
- Patients may experience the need to strain when having a bowel movement, and may also have pain during or after movement
- Constipation is common
- In severe cases, complete or partial incontinence, either faecal or urinary
- Sensation of having foreign object sitting inside vagina or rectum.

In France (Labat et al 2008), the Nantes criteria was published, where a consensus of 30 doctors working in this field established the diagnostic criteria for Pudendal Neuralgia by pudendal nerve entrapment.

The five essential criteria are

- Pain in the anatomical territory of the pudendal nerve
- Worsened by sitting
- The patient is not woken at night by the pain
- No objective sensory loss on clinical examination
- Positive anaesthetic pudendal nerve block.

Diagnosis

This is actually quite difficult and involves ruling out other possible causes, such as Coccydynia, Piriformis syndrome, Interstitial Cystitis, Myofascial trigger points (pelvic floor), Sacro-iliac joint dysfunction, Lumbar Radiculopathy

MRI scan may rule out prolapsed discs or pelvic tumours, but does not show nerve entrapment

EMG: Electromyography- trans-vaginal and also rectal; this is an electrical recording of muscle activity that aids the diagnosis of neuromuscular disease

Diagnostic pudendal nerve block can be confirmatory at either ischial spine level or Alcock's canal level. If there is some temporary relief of pain following one of these types of nerve block, it appears to indicate there may be a degree of nerve entrapment, which may benefit from surgical decompression surgery.

MRN scan: There is a form of Magnetic Resonance Imaging (MRI), called Magnetic Resonance Neurography that has been developed by a neurosurgeon from the USA. It is a nerve imaging technology that is similar to an MRI scan, but is finely tuned to highlight nerves. Magnetic Resonance Neurography is used to evaluate major nerve compressions such as those affecting the pudendal nerve, sciatic nerve or virtually any named nerve in the body. Unfortunately, these scans are only available at a high cost, around £800, and although they have been in use for fifteen years, some insurance companies may still classify this as experimental and decline to reimburse payment. This neurosurgeon does visit London approximately every 6 weeks, but an hour long consultation to follow up the scan may also prove quite costly.

Chapter 5 -
Treatments

In the first three sections of this chapter on the available treatments, I will be describing my own experiences with these treatments. I have tried various "nerve pain" medications and have undergone numerous nerve blocks, with very little benefit and have tried manual physiotherapy. When we come to the latter three sections, this information is what I have researched myself, or have been advised by others from the Pelvic Pain Support Network and form part of the normal treatment algorithm for pudendal neuralgia, (but are not so far part of my own experience). In the physiotherapy section, I have taken some information from the pelvicphysiotherapy.com web site managed by a group of physiotherapists who practice this specialist "hands on" technique. As I have now experienced this form of treatment, I am also able now to speak first hand.

Drug Therapy

Due to my background as an informed Health Professional,

I was able to recognize the pain that I experienced was probably "Nerve Pain", and so knew that conventional painkillers were of little value. I think this may have assisted me in making more rapid progress through the maze of consultants, as I understood a little better what might be going on.

Amitryptiline This was the first drug I was prescribed (a tricyclic antidepressant) and is known for its' positive benefits when treating pelvic nerve pain. As it also has quite a sedative effect at higher doses, it is important that the drug is started at the lowest possible dose-10mg, due to the sedatory impact. At this dose I could tolerate the drug, but by the time I had gradually increased the dose to 25mgs, I had an intensely itchy rash appearing all over the trunk of my body. I started taking Piriton 4mg to try and relieve the symptoms, but the itching rash became unbearable and my GP told me to stop taking the Amitryptiline, as I was probably allergic to it. The tricyclic group, are well known for their properties of addressing nerve pain, although it is outside of their licence to use in this way. Imipramine, which is in the same class of drugs, can also be used in the same way as Amitryptiline.

Pregabalin This drug should be started at a low dose, initially 150mg/day in 2 or 3 divided doses. It then needs to be increased to 300mg/day in divided doses, or even gradually to a maximum of 600mg/day. I was started at a low dose and had to try and increase the dose gradually, until I reached a minimum therapeutic dose (300mg daily). I started on 25mg, then 50mg, then 100mg, by then my sleep was regularly disturbed, and I felt quite woozy much of the time, particularly when I woke and seemed to have lost strength in my limbs, so that I found it a tremendous struggle even to walk. I kept dropping the dose and then trying to increase it again knowing that this low dose would be insufficient to improve the nerve pain symptoms (i.e. not therapeutically effective). As the dose I needed was 300mg/day, I soon realized that I could never reach that, and was not sure that at the low dose I took, there could be any really beneficial effect.

Pregabalin is one of a group of drugs primarily used to treat epilepsy, but also found to help with nerve pain, and along with others such as Gabapentin, is often used to help patients suffering from neuropathic pain due to diabetes. Gabapentin (which is much less expensive than Pregabalin) had according to my GP the potential for more unpleasant side effects than the Pregabalin, so he decided it was not worth me trying that. Again, it has been interesting to learn since then, that patients vary greatly in whether they develop more side effects from Gabapentin or from Pregabalin. Both these drugs are recommended by NICE for the treatment of neuropathic pain. Gabapentin, too can be prescribed for epilepsy, but is recognized as effective in treating nerve pain. The first Pain Management Consultant wanted me to continue taking the Pregabalin, whilst he tried various other treatment options, as he didn't want to alter the starting point. Later in my course of treatments I was also prescribed Gabapentin, but started falling asleep during the day whilst driving, even on the lowest dose.

Tramadol After the steroid injection into my urethra, the anaesthetist commenced me on Tramadol, for pain, as I required something to help control the pain. I was reluctant to start taking this, as it is an opioid agonist and may become addictive. I was glad that I tried it, as I found it to be the only effective pain relief; but as before I could only tolerate a small dose once every 24 hours, as it would make me very drowsy (in combination with the Pregabalin), and at times I nearly fell asleep driving home from work. I persisted with it, at an absolute minimum dose of 1x50mg/day, because it was the one analgesia that I tried that actually gave me relief for a few hours, unlike anything else. I then discovered, that it is documented by experts that Tramadol does help nerve pain, unlike such things as the anti-inflammatory group of drugs, Paracetamol and the Codeine combinations. I have now been taking Tramadol almost every day for well over a year, but really feel I am left with little option. Since stopping the pregabalin I have been able to increase the dose of Tramadol to 100mg once or twice a day when necessary.

It is important to recognize which drugs are effective in helping nerve pain, rather than spend time taking drugs that are of little or no benefit, and may even cause untoward side effects.

Oxycodone As I could only initially tolerate Tramadol in such small doses, this synthetic opioid, was then prescribed in the summer. However, this drug, even at low doses made me seriously drowsy, and had no impact on the pain (I obviously stopped taking the Tramadol for this period). As I could not increase the dose due to its' drowsiness effect I had to give up the Oxycodone and return to the Tramadol. This is another drug that can be effective against nerve pain, but my metabolism could not cope with it.

Duloxetine In late November 2009, the uro-genital pain specialist suggested that I try this drug, really as a temporary measure, until he could carry out the nerve block under CT scan mid January 2010. As he was aware that I seemed to be very sensitive to so many drugs, he prescribed 30mg/day (half the minimum dose for nerve pain). It is a newer drug than some of the others I had tried, but as nothing so far had made any real impact, I was keen to give this a go.

The National Institute for Health and Clinical Excellence (NICE) recommend Duloxetine as a gold standard for treating diabetic neuropathy. It also has therapeutic value as an anti depressant, which for me was a bonus, as it meant I did not have to take the additional anti depressant (Citalopram), which my own GP had just prescribed.

Soon after I commenced the Duloxetine, I felt so nauseated that I could hardly eat, so dropped to alternate days, but by the following weekend, there was no resolution to the nausea, so I had to find something to relieve this problem. I bought some Domperidone (an anti emetic) over the counter, from the local pharmacist, and on the next Monday, went to my GP and requested a prescription for the same. In that initial period, due to the nausea I lost half a stone in weight, and found I had little energy to do what I would normally do. I then tried taking the Duloxetine every day for about 10 days, and it had a really good effect on the nerve pain. In fact I hadn't felt this pain free, for well over a year, and I was almost able to stop taking any Tramadol for a week or so, however, I still felt incredibly nauseated.

In the end I tried reducing the Duloxetine to alternate days again to see how effective that was and then try increasing the number of consecutive days I could tolerate the drug. For the first few days I was fine, covered by what I had taken so far, then the pain started coming back and I was back to taking Tramadol almost every day. After 2 weeks at this level I increased to taking Duloxetine two days out of every three, this did make an improvement, and the level of the pain was not like it had been before I had tried taking this drug.

I was unable to increase the dose any more, as, my metabolism did not seem to tolerate the normal therapeutic dose, which is in fact 60mg/day, the maximum dose being 120mg/day.

Despite the draw-backs with Duloxetine, it had a beneficial effect on the pain, and enabled me to maintain some sort of normal life for a few months.

Fluoxetine (Prozac) Unfortunately, during the past summer months, one of the side effects from Duloxetine of extreme drowsiness seemed to take over, and made driving rather hazardous. This meant another change in nerve pain medication. My GP wisely advised me not to go for the Imipramine, as it is very likely to make me drowsy as well, so I tried Fluoxetine- more commonly known as Prozac (this had been recommended by the London specialist, if I was unable to tolerate the duloxetine). I am currently trying the Prozac as it gives me very few untoward side effects, to see if it is effective in helping to manage the pain. This drug appears to have assisted in reducing the pain and thankfully I have been able to tolerate taking Prozac, although there are some effects which I would like to be rid of, so I look forward in the future to possibly trying to reduce the dose, if the Physiotherapy brings enough of an improvement. By the time this book is published I am hopeful that I may have been able to reduce or even stop both the Tramadol and the Prozac.

Other Drugs: There are other drugs, which have been used to try and help with nerve pain, but many seem to carry a variety of challenging side effects. Each individual seems to respond slightly differently to each of the drugs, and it appears very difficult to predict what may or may not work. Drug therapy needs to be carefully monitored, due to the combined effects of several drugs on the body, and the ongoing impact of taking any drugs for the long-term.

In the area of drug therapy and balancing out the drugs available, it is important to try different combinations, if certain ones don't have any real benefit, or cause too many undesirable side- effects. There are several tricyclic drugs, which work in the same ways as the Amitryptiline, one of them being Imipramine; likewise with the Pregabalin there are others such as Gabapentin which can also be considered. Duloxetine is a gold standard drug in the treatment of Diabetic neuropathy, but if it is not tolerable, Venlafaxine in a similar group of anti depressants may give a similar benefit and also Fluoxetine.

Nerve Block Interventions

Here, I will describe the nerve blocks I have experienced and hopefully this will enable others to consider the best route to suit their particular needs.

In order for these to have any chance of being effective, it is important to obtain an accurate diagnosis. Unfortunately, my first pain consultant, was unable to pinpoint which the actual nerve was that was causing my particular nerve pain problem. So, he used qualified guesswork instead, having heard my symptoms and description of the pain and what triggered it. Firstly he tried an epidural injection plus an inguinal nerve block, these appeared to make no significant difference at all, apart from the immediate local anaesthetic effect. It is my belief, that most people by the time they read a book such as this, will have been under the care of numerous health care professionals, and may well have had similar experiences to this.

A nerve block may be carried out under sedation; both of the consultants whom I saw used sedation, believing that even under sedation patients can respond when spoken to and indicate whether the needle used is touching a nerve. Other schools of thought, such as Nantes keep their patients completely awake during such a procedure, believing that this is better in assessing any immediate effect of the local anaesthetic and steroid. Local anaesthetic (normally Lidocaine) is injected onto the nerve concerned, under X-ray imaging using fluoroscopy (injection of contrast medium). This is done under these conditions to ensure precise placement of the needle, so that only the target nerve is affected. The needle used in these instances, is a fine 25mm gauge needle. Following this a steroid is injected onto the particular nerve. Initially the local anaesthetic reduces the pain felt, and then within 10 days or so after the procedure, the steroid effect should reduce the nerve inflammation and thereby also the pain experienced.

In my experience, this was all done as a day case procedure, with someone available to take me home following the procedure due to the effects of the sedation. The second procedure I underwent, was a Ganglion Impar Block. A ganglion impar is where a bunch of nerves clusters together, in the lower back; this cluster is situated in front of the joint between the sacrum and coccyx. This procedure was carried out under similar conditions to the previous nerve block, and seemed to produce a mild improvement for a few days. In view of this, the pain specialist believed that maybe he had found the source of the pain, and decided to go a stage further and stun the nerves electrically- this is called radio-frequency denervation. (In this procedure extreme heat is used, by placing the probe close to the affected nerve and radio waves used to generate extreme heat through the tip for 40-90 seconds.) This normally completes what the steroid injection began and reduces the nerve irritation; however for me it stirred up the pain response from the nerves, so could not be repeated.

This type of nerve block is reported (Foye 2006), to provide good pain relief, reducing pain felt by 50-75% in those with a Coccydynia type of pain. Mine was obviously not Coccydynia, as it did not respond in this way.

I was then transferred to the uro- genital pain consultant, who recommended a course of 3 nerve block injections at the levels of the ischial spines. As the pain appeared to be on both sides, I had bilateral nerve blocks. These were all conducted as with the initial nerve blocks, under sedation (not anaesthetic), and under X-ray imaging guidance (fluoroscopy), to pinpoint the nerves precisely. The local anaesthetic is then injected on the nerve to numb the area and then the steroid is injected onto the nerves on both sides each time. The first had a marginal effect for a day or so, but the subsequent two appeared to change nothing.

I was then booked for further nerve blocks on both sides again at the level of Alcock's canal, carried out under CT scan guidance, as Alcock's canal is deeper internally and needs more careful isolation of the nerves. Although after the first of these I stated that I did not want any more, I was informed that if I subsequently transferred to the National Health Service (NHS) for any further pain management, the first procedure they would most likely carry out would be a nerve block at the Alcock's Canal level if I did not have the 2nd block at this point. It seemed sensible therefore, to go ahead, as advised with the second nerve block at this level. Unfortunately, this final nerve block, instead of suppressing the pain, actually triggered a pain flare up for about 2-3 weeks following the procedure, so I wished I had stuck to my original intentions.

However, having had a total of 5 Pudendal Nerve blocks, I have since been informed that the maximum number of nerve blocks that the Nantes team of pain management doctors will carry out is three. At the Convergences in Pelvic-Perineal Pain congress in December 2009 there was a request that this should in fact be just two. One nerve block would be done at the level of the Ischial spine and the other at the Alcock's canal level. (It is worth noting that the ischial spine injections carried out in Nantes are via the buttock and CT guided and there are some other differences in how they carry out these procedures, which may explain the different success rates between them and other experts). It is worth noting that there are various ways of carrying out nerve blocks with both advantages and disadvantages.

Pudendal Nerve Blocks may be used both as a diagnostic tool and a treatment procedure; and normally, if the nerve block produces any temporary relief of pain, however short, this normally is an indication that the pain is pudendal in origin. I experienced only marginal improvement with the first of the pudendal nerve blocks, and all my symptoms seem to be consistent with pudendal nerve damage symptoms. The consultant's opinion was that the nerve damage was too severe, which is why I did not respond positively to the blocks, and so nerve decompression surgery would probably be of no benefit to me. I was left feeling very disappointed on hearing this. Again, this is not necessarily the interpretation different experts may give at this point as others who have had surgery have suggested to me.

Pain Psychology

In the treatment of chronic pain such as Pudendal Neuralgia, it has long been considered that Pain Psychology and Cognitive Behavioural Therapy (CBT) have a role in enabling the patient to manage their pain, and whilst not removing the pain, helping the person to find ways of coping. The reason for encouraging CBT is that it is quite rare for complete or sustained remission to be obtained in treating chronic pain of any sort. The aim of treatment is to reduce the suffering and improve quality of life. CBT may well assist patients in managing their response to pain more positively, so that they can cope from day to day. This has been recommended to me, and as I have heard that people have benefitted from this approach, it is definitely something I will consider and I would suggest that if you are someone who is currently struggling to come to terms with chronic nerve pain caused by pudendal neuralgia, then please don't dismiss it.

Pain psychologists can help with developing strategies to cope with or manage the pain; they are also skilled at helping to separate the depression and anxiety from the pain itself, so that it becomes possible to stop the roller coaster of emotions that constantly threaten as pain intensity varies. This is again something that I have experienced, and know the need for something to help break the cycle.

Cognitive Behaviour Therapy helps, by retraining thought patterns, and challenging negative thoughts and feelings, which are quite obviously going to be part of a cycle of chronic pain. It can help in breaking down the problem into smaller components. There are probably 4 keys aspects:

1. The specific problems are identified; here they will be related to the experience of pain, and an attempt is made to solve them
2. Goals are set, which need to be achieved, to address the specific problems
3. It is concerned with how we think and act now

4. Provides a partnership and support to work out with the therapist how to improve the situation.

The following is a summary of some of the key ways that pain psychology may help someone with chronic pain:

- Provide support and help in problem solving
- Teach skills that may decrease pain levels
- Assist in discerning what activities may be helpful and what should be avoided.
- Figure out which individual coping skills are useful and which may in fact hinder coping with the pain
- Prescribe medication, which may decrease pain or increase ability to handle your situation
- Aid in evaluating whether there is depression or anxiety that contributes to the pain
- Address any problem with sleep (this problem sometimes occurs with some of the nerve pain medicines.

Hopefully, this very brief summary of how psychology can really benefit chronic pain sufferers may help those of you reading this to have an open mind in asking for support of this kind, or being ready to embrace this kind of therapy.

Physiotherapy

The physiotherapy route, seems to have several approaches, one is a hands-on or manual technique the other a hands-off approach. The latter consists mainly of stretching exercises and is seen by some as more limited. Currently there are only a handful of physiotherapists practicing manual therapy in the UK, and who have the appropriate training or experience to help people like myself with pudendal nerve pain, so it is very difficult to find such a physiotherapist. These therapists are mainly private practitioners, and they are not always available under health insurance cover. However, there are a number in the UK who are accessible.

Manual therapy involves the process of physically releasing tight muscles that will not let go voluntarily. The patient may eventually be able to perform their own manual therapy themselves after training from the therapist. However it is preferable, that manual therapy be carried out, in the first instance by an appropriately trained physiotherapist. Specialist training is necessary for physiotherapists to use manual therapy in treating such conditions as Pudendal Neuralgia. Not only will the therapists need a strong bias towards manual therapy but also an extensive working knowledge of the condition.

This technique may include stretching and trigger point treatment, where a muscle is tense. This problem can be identified by internal examination and then stretched centrally along the bulk of the muscle or at the attachment to bone, which can be more uncomfortable. Trigger points will frequently refer pain elsewhere in the pelvic floor, or to the hips or rectum, or may in fact be painful at the spot itself. Once held for a few seconds the pain eases and the therapist can move on to the next point. The nerves in the pelvic floor can also be mobilised along their pathways.

Manual therapy should not be so painful that the patient tenses up in response to it and the pelvic floor muscles should not be sore following manual therapy. Therapy is very individual, and will be tailored by the physiotherapist to meet the needs of each patient. For more information about manual therapy and the therapists who practise it, see the following website: www.pelvicphysiotherapy.com.

At the pain management centre I attended in London, the approach to physiotherapy is mainly hands off, where the physiotherapist will supply a range of exercises for the patient to work on, to reduce muscle spasm in the affected region. The hands on approach, may seem more invasive in some senses, but tackles the muscle spasm directly, initially using the professional's digits at trigger points to relieve spasm (as described earlier), and then the patient can be taught to do this for themselves, or have the help of a spouse or partner to do it for them.

A friend, whom I have got to know through the pelvic pain support network, has had some months of manual therapy. She strongly recommends this type of treatment, as she would say that she has had a 70% improvement in the pain she experiences and has been able to reduce considerably the amount of medication she needs to take in order to control the pain. This personal recommendation stimulated me to ask my GP to refer me to a specialist physiotherapist for manual therapy. At my first appointment, I was assessed thoroughly by this physiotherapist and a comprehensive history of the pain also taken. She believed that there were ways in which she could help to improve my situation. I used the pelvic-physiotherapy website to find suitably qualified therapists. There are such physiotherapists working in the NHS, but I was informed by one of them that the waiting lists are quite long.

I have stopped having Manual Therapy now, because the pain returned despite the treatment with the physiotherapist, and initially, because some of the pelvic floor muscles were so contracted I found my pain was aggravated by the therapy. Initially I noticed a reduction in the pain I experienced and hoped it would continue. I am aware that this sort of treatment may again seem undignified, but when one experiences a marked reduction of the pain, particularly in its' intensity, I believe it is worth the indignity. The whole condition has been difficult to discuss and describe, so a period of further vulnerability for appropriate treatment, with an understanding practitioner was not a problem for me. In fact I felt little embarrassment at the time as care was taken to protect both my privacy and dignity. At later sessions, biofeedback was used to help in improving the contraction and relaxation of my pelvic floor muscles; unfortunately this triggered more severe pain and therefore was not used again.

The aim of both therapies is to minimize or eliminate the concurrent pain generators that occur when the pudendal nerve is irritated. This may be in the form of increased muscle tone, or very tense muscle and myofascial trigger points, extra pelvic increased muscle tone and trigger points, adverse nerve tension, sacro-iliac joint dysfunctions and faulty neuromuscular recruitment patterns, as well as connective tissue restrictions. This link between musculoskeletal and nerve dysfunction needs to be acknowledged, as it is rather unusual to have one existing without the other. This all sounds rather technical and complex, but in simple terms it relates to over contracted or over tense muscles, which may then trap or press on nerves in various places, causing the pain. They may then cause a cycle of pain to be established and somehow, through this manual therapy, the aim is to break this pattern and restore normal muscle tone. At times, the pain is aggravated by the therapy, but the overall trend is one of improvement.

Decompression Surgery

For those who have suffered the intense pain of Pudendal Neuralgia for a number of years, decompression surgery offers a real hope of improvement. From questions I have posed on the Pelvic Pain Network message board the answers I have received, speak very highly about people's experiences of treatment in Nantes. They are so pleased with the care they have received in Nantes. Most of those who have surgery will probably go to Nantes, as it is the centre of excellence for this aspect of medicine. Some patients are able to obtain funding from the NHS, through application to their local Primary Care Trust, others may pay for the consultations and treatment themselves, out of an intense desperation caused by the nature of the pain.

However, there is now a surgeon carrying out this surgery in London, although his experience does not extend as far back as the team from Nantes. The team in Nantes have been performing decompression surgery since 1987, whilst the London surgeon started much more recently. Professor Robert, a member of the team in Nantes pioneered one of the approaches to surgical decompression, which is the "Trans-gluteal" approach. Patients, who have treatment in Nantes, normally undergo pudendal nerve blocks first to assess their response and suitability for decompression surgery.

Nerve healing takes time, but those people who I have had contact with, say that they become gradually aware that they are able to do more than they were and are not so limited by the pain. Some say that the pain is reduced by as much as 60 -70 % over a few years following surgery.

For those who are older, surgery may not be an option, as the healing process can be considerably slower. Also, the length of time the symptoms have existed and the extent that the nerves are affected will also influence the decision of the surgeon as to whether surgery is the best option.

Surgical approaches

1. The "Trans Gluteal" approach, where the Pudendal nerve is visualized in order to surgically decompress or release it as necessary. This is done through an incision to the buttocks on both sides.
2. The Transperineal Approach, which is via a para-anal incision. The disadvantage of this method is that the procedure is limited by its small area of exposure and incomplete access to all possible areas of entrapment.
3. Trans-ischio-rectal approach:

For women, this involves a vertical vaginal incision, where the para-rectal space is entered

For men, a para median transverse perineal incision is made and then the para-rectal space is entered.

The disadvantages of this latter method, is again the smaller field of vision available for the procedure, and also expertise is required in intra operative nerve testing. One of its advantages is that it avoids direct manipulation of the nerve, thus reducing the risk of nerve damage surgically.

Margaret Stubbs

Sacral Root Stimulation

This involves the surgical insertion of electrical wires into the sacral nerve root of the spine. These wires then interrupt the nerve pain impulses and reduce the pain experienced. This procedure has been performed since 1988 for bladder and bowel instability. This treatment is available on the NHS. The spinal cord stimulator is a procedure that has been recognized by the National Institute for Health and Clinical Excellence as a valid treatment for chronic pain and the sacral root stimulator operates in a similar way. The way the stimulator works, is that it is a small battery powered device that is designed to deliver precise amounts of electricity to your spinal cord; this then alters the way in which pain signals are processed and can have a dramatic effect on pain in some people.

Initially, temporary wires are inserted, this may be done under sedation and there is a trial period of several days. This is done to ensure that the system is reducing the pain experienced by a fair percentage, and also because the permanent device costs over £10,000, and so care needs to be taken, to make sure it suits the person concerned. Application has to be made to the appropriate Primary Care Trust for funding for this equipment. If the trial is successful and funding available, then a permanent device may be inserted, and surgery under a general anaesthetic is required to install the components. The device is made up of the stimulating system, which is positioned in the abdomen or side of the chest, the electrodes, which are positioned near the spinal cord, and then there is a lead, which connects the two parts of the device. Apparently, concern has been expressed at the International Convergences Pelvic Pain congress about the possible use of this to treat a nerve, which may be entrapped. Currently it is a last resort in the treatment algorithm after surgery along with intrathecal pain pumps.

Botox Injections

Very little seems to be known about the use of Botox injection for helping with pain. However, a few people have stated that they have received these injections and they obtained relief for as much as 6 months. In France and Australia, the pain management consultants have used Botox Injections, but it is generally not available in the UK. Its' use has not been recorded recently, although there have been reported cases within the past ten years of a few patients receiving Botox injections in the UK for relief of pain. Its impact is mainly on the muscular pain component.

Botox, is in fact not licensed for this purpose in the UK. In Australia it is at the patient's own expense.

Research

New treatments are being developed to help with the management of nerve pain of this type. Currently a randomized controlled trial of different types of nerve blocks is underway in several centres in France.

Chapter 6 -
Chronic Pain versus Acute Pain

In seeking to come to terms with this chronic nerve pain, it is important to understand the key differences between acute and chronic pain. There is also the need to understand that nerve pain is different from nociceptive pain. Nociceptive pain occurs when there is injury or damage to parts of the body, and the nociceptors are the nerves, which send and respond to the parts of the body suffering the damage. It is also time limited, meaning that when the tissue damage heals the pain will resolve. This type of pain responds well to treatment with opioid drugs.

Nerve pain is not necessarily about damage or injury to an organ in the body or a limb; rather the pain comes as result of damaged nerves, either that have been compressed or damaged in some way sending out the wrong messages so that this nerve pain is then experienced. The pain may have been triggered by an injury, but this injury may or may not involve actual damage to the nervous system. Pain may not always be just neuropathic or nociceptive, there may from time to time be a combination of the two types occurring side by side in the same person. The treatment may involve disrupting these nerve/brain signals so that pain is not felt (Richeimer 2000). Myofascial pain is an example of this, it is probably secondary to the nociceptive input from the muscles, but there is abnormal muscle activity, which may have resulted from a neuropathic condition.

Nerve pain is frequently chronic and tends to respond less well to opioid drug treatment. It is not normally fully reversible, but with appropriate treatment partial improvement is possible.

Chronic pain is defined in a huge variety of ways, and these are just some of the definitions that I have come across:

> *"Pain that may range from mild to severe and persists or progresses over a long period of time"*

> *" Chronic pain is a state in which pain persists beyond the usual course of an acute disease or healing of an injury"*

> *" A pain state, which is persistent and in which the cause of the pain cannot always be removed or is difficult to treat. Chronic pain may be associated with a long term incurable or intractable medical condition or disease"*

A popular and acceptable definition is:

> *"Pain that extends beyond the expected period of healing"*

There is disagreement about whether pain becomes chronic after 3 or after 6 months, but in general it is agreed that it is long term and hard to treat. This pain also tends to have significant psychological and emotional effects on the person and limits the person's ability to fully function.

It is recognized that chronic pain causes other symptoms or conditions such as depression and anxiety. It seems that there has been little work done on the cognitive effects of chronic pain. Most publications have looked at the effects of cognition on pain, but only 5% have examined the effects of pain on cognition and mental functioning. Chronic pain affects the ability to direct attention. In tests (Dick 2007) that have been carried out, individuals with the highest levels of pain show greater disruption of memory traces, suggesting that pain may diminish working memory.

People with high intensity chronic pain have (C Eccleston 1995), it is suggested a significantly reduced ability to perform attention demanding tasks. It would appear (A Von Bueren Jarchow et al 2005) that pain sensations dominate the attention of people with chronic pain, so that they may demonstrate poorer performance than their peers who do not experience chronic pain, on all sorts of tests, which demand attention.

Although, all this has to be recognized, it should not be forgotten that whilst sustained remission of neuropathic and chronic pain is rarely experienced, there are a number of things that can be done to reduce the suffering and improve the quality of life. I have tried to outline in the earlier section on treatments, the different ways of learning to manage pain. What I believe is key to managing this type of chronic nerve pain is to know that there is support from others available, places to go for advice, suggestions of new therapies that work for some and not for others. It is vital to be aware that as individuals, we are not alone in all this and there are other people to talk to. Through the Pelvic Pain Support Network I have found other people like myself, who either have experienced or still experience similar pain and have gone down varying treatment pathways and are helping others to find ways of managing their pain more effectively.

Part of the process of coming to terms with long term pain, is being able to acknowledge that life goes on, but in a modified format. If this means carrying certain pieces of equipment around to make sitting more bearable, and having to limit certain activities to minimise the pain and its impact, then this is all part of the process. At the same time, one has to keep looking for possible alternatives to bring the pain under control or subdue it. For myself, this means finding the right balance between activity and rest, and not being afraid to admit that I have a chronic pain problem, as it is amazing what openings this sometime provides. For me it has also involved giving up a favourite hobby, cycling.

It can also entail having to adjust to different working days in order to manage the pain, or resting when there are friends or family around. This can be very challenging at times, for someone like myself, who likes to lead a full and active life, and would like to achieve at a high level where possible.

However what it does not mean is giving up on life and just accepting the pain, but finding alternative ways of doing things. The options of acupuncture, chiropractic and osteopathy, massage, hydrotherapy are all alternative ways of attempting to relieve chronic pain. There are also other alternative means of managing chronic pain, which I may not have mentioned. There may not be a lot of evidence to support all these approaches, but they can be worth trying, as different approaches may provide benefit for different people, just as drugs can have varying impacts on individuals.

Chapter 7 -
Aids to Assist Normal Living

As sitting is one of the most uncomfortable positions with pudendal neuralgia, it is vital to have equipment to assist with this. One of the key reasons to sit correctly, is that sitting with legs tucked underneath the body and to one side (sometimes referred to as "picnic style") creates a very poor posture, so that hips and spine may became deformed and this then leads to pressure on intevertebral discs and causes other nerve pain, or muscular spasm as the other muscles in the back try to compensate in this position. This then becomes an additional problem to the neuralgia, and one that needs to be avoided. An obvious alternative to sitting, is to stand for short periods to relieve the pressure from sitting, or to do things lying down as well, which is perfectly possible with the use of lap top computers.

A very simple, but effective aid is a foam cushion in the shape of a toilet seat, with the centre cut out; this is confirmed by the number of sufferers who say that sitting on a toilet seat is the most comfortable way of sitting down. Basically this is therefore a thick foam ring, cut to support the shape of the person's buttocks, with the centre being cut out. The ring is then mounted on a thick card base behind the centre hole, and then covered with a stretchy fabric. This then becomes like a portable and also soft "toilet" type seat, with no pressure on the perineal area, which is so sensitive to resting on anything for very long. It is even relatively easy to carry around, to restaurants or theatres, if trying to be more ambitious. It is also quite durable, I have had mine for almost two years now and carry it round all over the place, so that I can attend work related meetings or meetings on behalf of the Pelvic Pain Support Network, and keep up with some of my interests outside of the home.

A second piece of equipment, which has proved useful, is the kneeling chair; these chairs are actually designed for those with back problems, to ensure a better posture when sitting down doing almost anything from computer work, to reading, to handicrafts. Here the majority of weight and pressure is carried in the knees, relieving the perineal areas. These chairs come at a variety of prices and can be quite costly; the key to finding a good one, does involve trying them out. These vary also as to how long a period of time one can use them before needing to move around for a while, but again they reduce bad posture and the other complications that may develop from that. Many providers of equipment for those with back problems will be able to supply these as well as suppliers of office equipment, such as Staples, (www.staples.co.uk for information about both stock and delivery), prices start at £54.99.

Another help, which I obviously can only advise female sufferers about, is underwear. This seems to vary as a problem, but for me, underwear has become a real problem. I find that when the pain is particularly bad, I cannot wear underwear with seams, as the seams give the sensation of being rubbed or cut into two along the perineum. I have had to invest in seamless underwear for any such occasion, and also for later in the day when the pain increases. At the moment I am ordering this from the USA, but as importation duty is sometime charged, I am looking for an alternative in the UK. My current supplier is www.freshpair.com.

It is worth considering the place of heat and or ice in helping to manage the pain. I have found heat to be useful, whereas there are others who think ice works better to ease the discomfort experienced.

Chapter 8 -
Conclusion

In conclusion, I want to reiterate that this book is aimed at trying to help fellow sufferers come to terms with their chronic nerve pain, and know where to find support and help to do this. There may be new treatments and therapies available as time goes on which may bring more lasting relief than is currently possible and I want to do all in my power to not only access that, but make sure that everyone else with a similar condition, knows how to access the appropriate therapy that will provide the best benefit for them as an individual.

I have tried to make this book readable by the average layperson and not a technical handbook for use by pain specialists. There are a few technical books written by pain management experts, but they do not address the issues from a perspective of experience with this type of pain. However there are a couple of books which friends with pudendal neuralgia have recommended. The first is: Headache in The Pelvis written by David Wise and Rodney Anderson. This book is primarily aimed at men, but does give some insight into the muscles that contribute to pelvic pain. The second book is: Explain Pain, which is written by David Butler and Lorimer Moseley, and is a book, which deals in detail with the whole subject of pain.

I have personally tried several of the available treatments for pudendal neuralgia, and with the initially positive experience with the Manual Therapy, I would say this is the one to have produced the most significant benefits for me. Obviously, different treatments may not be as effective in each individual, but this I have found to be such a bonus. Also, I have valued good friendships more than ever since this pain entered my life, and the support of friends and family makes so much difference. On a lighter note, I have learnt to talk with less embarrassment about the more private parts of my body and also with close family and friends find some humour, learning not to take myself too seriously all the time.

If, I can be of assistance to anyone reading this book who may be currently struggling with pelvic nerve pain of any sort, please feel free to contact me, via the pelvic pain network. But whatever you do, don't give up, there are a number of treatments for this most embarrassing of problems now, and make sure you get referred to the appropriate expert, so that you received the best help and support. It is important to go through the less invasive options first, and try them out, before embarking on the more invasive ones such as Spinal Cord Stimulation or Decompression surgery.

I would like to thank those fellow sufferers who have read through this manuscript for me to check for inaccuracies, and advised me accordingly. I hope this book will be of help to many.

Helpful websites

www.pelvicpain.org.uk: support network for anyone with any type of pelvic pain, not solely pudendal nerve pain

www.spuninfo.org: The Society for Pudendal Neuralgia

www.action-on-pain.co.uk; deals with all types of pain

www.painconcern.org.uk; again, this addresses all types of pain and how to manage chronic pain

www.britishpainsociety.org.uk: national organisation working on behalf of patients with all types of pain

www.pelvicphysiotherapy.com: for further advice and information about manual therapy; contact details of the therapists and exercises to help relieve muscle tension

www.painassociation.com: for self- management programmes

www.patients-association.org.uk: helping patients in every area of healthcare, with their needs

www.paincoalition.org.uk: organisation fighting for the needs of patients with chronic pain; putting chronic pain on the health care agenda

www.vulvalpainsociety.org.uk: this organisation is concerned with all types of vulval pain and not just that caused by pudendal neuralgia

www.freshpair.com; seam free underwear

www.staples.co.uk: kneeling chairs

References

Dick B D & Rashiq S (2007) Disruption of attention and working memory traces in individuals with chronic pain. *Anaesthesia Analgesia* **104**(5): 1223-1229

Eccleston C (1995) Chronic pain and distraction: an experimental investigation into the role of sustained and shifting attention in the process of chronic persistent pain *Behaviour Research Therapy* **33**(4): 391-405

J J Labat, T Riant et al (2008) Diagnostic Criteria for Pudendal Neuralgia by Pudendal Nerve Entrapment *Neurology and Urodynamics* **27**(4): 306-310

Richeimer S (2000) The Richeimer Pain Update from the Richeimer Pain Medical Group December 2000

Von Bueren Jarchow A, Radanov B P, Jancke l (2005). Pain influences several levels of attention *Zeitschrift fur Neuropsychologie*

www.Howtocopewithpain.org; Should I see a pain management Psychiatrist, Psychologist or Therapist?

Further Reading:

Headache in the Pelvis: David Wise and Rodney Anderson. Published by the National Centre for Pelvic Pain Research

Explain Pain: David Butler and Lorimer Moseley. Published by Notgroup Publication

About the Author

The author Margaret Stubbs is an experienced and well-qualified Practice Nurse with a Master's Degree in Primary Care. The majority of her life she has lived in the UK, where she has married and also raised three children. For most of her 50 years she has been in excellent health and it was only in late 2008 that the current problems began. The onset of pelvic nerve pain was triggered by minor bladder surgery.

The pain has affected every area of her life, particularly her working life, where adjustments have had to be made. However, despite this chronic pain, she endeavours to live as normal a life as possible, and most people are probably oblivious to the fact she has this pain. She believes that the combination of her nursing skills and knowledge and her current experience give her a unique understanding of this pain and the desire to help others through writing this book.